A-Z of Over 200 Diseases And Their Cures

ABDUL GANEEY YAQEEN FALOLA

First Published by Ib9ja Info-Tech Press

ISBN: 9781650907130

DEDICATION

All praises, adoration, adulation are due to none save God, the nourisher, the cherisher and the sustainer of the worlds, I beseech his help to send down his countless mercy upon the prophets, their house hold companions generality of Muslims.

An adage says "health is wealth". The compilation of A-Z of diseases and their cures is to please GOD ALMIGHTY, the giver of knowledge and to provide a simple and concise remedies to people's health. The first part of the book introduce you to some natural healings.

The other part brief names of those herbs in our common and international languages, Hausa, Igbo, Yoruba, English and 30 natural health advice. All these we involve ourselves to seek the pleasures of God almighty, the uncreated creator.

CONTENTS

ACKNOWLEDGMENTS

We all know health is wealth and our major aim is to show to the world that you don't have to exceed limit of god before getting healed. In addition, the herbs or grasses you are seeing every day, you calculate them to be weed and felt that they are not useful as classified "unwanted", they are the best to make our body healthy.

APPENDIX

Appendix has first aid? Add red oil with honey, a spoon 1hr before food. 3 times

a)   Cup of warm water, 5 spoon of black seed powder, 3 spoon of honey. To be taken 1hr before   breakfast and 1 before dinner.

b)   Mix a cup of khal, a cup of honey and little garlic. Warm the mixture. Take it twice daily.

c)   Gel from aloe Vera leaf, add grounded garlic. A spoon of the mixture into a glass cup of warm water. Once in a day.

d)   Epo iroko, Isu gbegbe, Eru Alamo. Cook all with omi ogi (corn fermented water). Drink twice daily

e)   Lemon, 1tomato, snail fluid. Crush and grind the tomato with lemon water and later add snail fluid with the mixture. Once in a day till the problem is over

f)   Eyin olobe; Taking this herbs by soaking in water could solve the problem

NOTE: Any of my drugs that has honey in them must be taken, is either 1hr before food or 1hr after food (Ulcer patient should avoid the use of khal and lime juice).

ANTI-POISON

a)   Garlic oil, olive oil, honey mix all with little water and drink all 3times

b)   Take a spoonful of olive oil constantly

c)   Garlic powder 1 table spoon, 1 tin of milk, little water, olive oil 2 spoon. Mix all and drink half glass 3 times daily

d)   Drink coconut water, it neutralizes effect of poison

e)   Grind charcoal and give the person without water

f)   Six bitter cola, 1 bottle of palm kernel oil, 5 spoon of honey mix in a cup of milk Take all.

ASTHMA

a)   Mix a bottle of honey, a cup of khal and a tin of habatu saudah powder. 2 spoons 3 times daily

b)   Rub khal tufa into the nostrils.

c)   Swallows a garlic after each meal.

d)   Pound garlic , mix with a bottle of honey. A spoon every 1hours, before every meal.

e)   Isumeric, Ori, Erualamo, Kerewu, cook all, a spoon for child.

f)   Rub the chest and back with black seed oil and 3 spoons oil per day.

ASTHMA COUGH IN CHILDREN

a)   Pound five bulbs of garlic, a bottle of saudah oil, 5 spoons of khal, a bottle of honey and half cup of orange juice. 2 spoons every 3 hours.

b)   Snail fluid, pure honey, same ratio and to be licked every 1 hour for 4-5 months. Snail fluid is blue in colour.

ASTHMA COUGH IN ADULT AND CHILDREN

5 Spoons of tumeric, 5 spoons of cinnamon powder mix with 1 ltr. bottle of honey. 2 spoons 2x daily after meal for 1 month. For baby 2spoons 2times daily.

ARTHRITIS

a)   Mix zaitun oil with Al- babunaj, boil the two and run on the affected part while it is still warm

b)   Mix four spoons of carrot juice, half cup of fresh cow milk, two spoons of honey drink daily for 2 months

c)   Pound aloe vera leaf with garlic fruits, mix with honey take it 3 times daily.

d)   Mix 1 tin of hulba powder, 1 tin of habatu saudah powder, 3 spoons of ginger powder, 1 bottle of garlic oil a spoon of cinnamon, 11 spoons of lime juice, half litre of honey, a cup of khal, 1 tin of turmeric powder, 2 spoons morning and evening after bathing with hot water, rub the affected part with zaitun oil mixed with habatu saudah oil lastly, do hijamah (cupping on the spot).

e)   5 Cloves of garlic, 5 worderful kola, 9 pieces of ginger,2 Roll of alligator pepper, 10 pieces of Iyere, 30g of Holy basil, 5 Pieces of Bitter kola, Lime juice, 10 Pieces of Turmeric, Moringa seeds. Pound all together and soak in a bottle of honey. 3 spoons morning and evening.

ANIMAL SICKNESS

Always put khal water, khal tufa, cinnamon into their bucket of drink water.

ALOPECIA (loss of Hair or Baldness)

a)	Mix chebe powder with zaitun oil (olive oil), rub on your head 3 times. It will stimulate hair growth

b)	Aloe vera, Black pepper, Indian hemp seed.blend it together in the same proportion massage twice daily

c)	Olive oil+Honey same quantity, warm it and apply on hair, after 30 minutes wash with warm water

d)	Dissolve **SHEA BUTTER**, Pound banana add aloe gel 3 spoons of honey, lemon juice 2 egg yolk, onion juice add all sieve, add to hair overnight,wash well to remove odour, add coconut and comb

ABDOMINAL PAIN

a)	Drink 3 spoons of zaitun oil in half cup of warm water 3 times daily.

b)	Soak 2 spoons of rashad powder in a cup of water, 1 spoon of lime juice into, drink all 3 times daily

c)	2 spoons of honey after meal till it stops 3 times

d)	Squeeze lime juice into half cup of warm water, and drink first thing in the morning for three.

e)	5ml full of salt in to a glass of water and mix &drink

f)	Bitter leaf (squeeze) together with palm oil 1 glass cup drink.

ANAEMIA

a)	Grind a handful of parsley leaves, Handful of cassava leaves, grind little ginger, squeeze out 1 lemon put the the mixture in a glass of honey. Add half litre of water and allow for 15 minutes mixing together, taking all within 3 days in the morning alone. Not more than 3 days

b)	Boil avocado leaves drink for a week

c)	Mix 6 tablespoons of tobacco leaves(dried powdered) in one bottle of honey 2 spoon 3 timed

ALCOHOLISM

a)	Large consumption of honey at a regular interval

APPETITE LOSS

a)	Grape fruit juice mixed with honey. Take at once

b)	15 minute before meal take 1 spoon of black seed oil

c)	Mix 2 spoons of aloe juice in orange juice twice daily

d)	A spoon of black seed powder a spoon of ginger powder, add to hot pap. Take it 2 days interval

e)	Brush your mouth with bitter leafs sticks.

BRAIN BOOSTER/SHARPNESS

a)	Always eat sebib in an empty stomach. Adult: 21 sebib before food, Kids: 7 sebib before food.

b)	Grind and mix the two together. Zukar nabat and luban zakar. Take a spoon of the mixture for two month with zamzam.

c)	Always give your kid honey right from birth till he or she reaches 5 years.

NOTE: BOTULISM SPORE occurs when there is dirt and dust in a honey and this could be dangerous to the new born.

d)	Boil nahana and habatu saudah powder. Take half cup every morning and rub your head with saudah oil.

e)	Slice a big fresh tomato, add a spoon a garlic powder, a spool of vinegar (Khal water), half spoon of salt. Eat all repeat it every day.

Get a coconut pour salt in it put it on fire and heat till you have it in powdery form. Use it to take pap.

BONE WEAKNESS IN CHILDREN

a)	When the child is up to $4^{1/2}$ month give him or her 3 spoons of carrot juice daily.

b)	Put habbatu saudah oil cold press in warm water and give him a spoon of the oil.

BODY TEMPERATURE

 Shower with cold water. Then take a spoon of saudah oil and also rub your body with it

BRONCHITIS

a)	Drink Guava leaves tea. Boil and drink

BREAST CANCER

a)	Honey and saudah seed

b)	Mix 4 cups of aloe Vera juice and a cup of honey. Take three spoon 3times daily.

c)	A tin of garlic powder, a tin of cress seed powder, 2 liters of honey with it wax, pineapple head. Take this mixture regularly.

d)	Pound a leaf of aloe Vera, rub the breast with it. Then wash it next day.

e)	15 fresh young sour sop leaf to 1 liter of water. Add little heat till that 1 liter of water reduces to half drink.

f)	1 aloe Vera, 1 pineapple, 1 sour sop fruit, 3 gingers. After remove the skins blend all. 1 cup morning & evening for 3 weeks

g)	Drink ewedu

h)	Mix camel milk with camel urine a spoon each.

BED WETTING (OLDER OR YOUNGER PERSON)

a)	Taking honey 1teaspoon 3 times daily but 2 spoons at bed time

b)	Buy diffusa powder and eat it with smoked yam for 3 days. God willing that is all.

c)	Habbatu saudah powder, luban zakar mix the two together an the person will take it with solid pap (eko) for seven days without missing a day. God willing it will go

d)	Get 4 big onions, squeeze out of the water in a cup. Mix with 4 small cups with 4 bottles of tulus water with khal water. Mix all 4 spoons 3 times daily

BIG BREAST (IF YOU DON'T HAVE BREAST AT ALL)

a)	Sun dry pandoro fruit and make into powder pandoro (kigelia) add into olive oil, use it to rub your chest

b)	Get marugbo roots, hulba powder, ajeobale leaves. Pound & sundry the two. Use it to take pap.

BOIL (EEWO) & BODY CRACK

a)	Wash the part with khal. Rub it with a mixture of zaitun and palmoil

b)	A tin of garlic powder, a bottle of honey, a bottle of zaitun oil 3 spoons every day.

c)	Do you know (SHIKITI) plants? It is the tiniest & smallest herbs of all leaves. It usually form carpet on the ground. Grind the leaves & add palm oil apply on the boil within 15 mins you see the miracle of God

BLEEDING NOSE

a)   Mix onion juice with khal (vinegar) soak a cotton wool in it,then put the wool into your nostrils.

b)   A spoon of onion juice, a spoon of honey, small lime juice be dropping it into the nose

BURN (Fire Incident)

a)   After the burn, apply khal.

b)   Wash the spot and apply honey.

c)   Rub aloe Vera on the spot 3 times daily.

d)   Habbata saudah, Zaitun oil, egg york. Apply on the spot

BONE & BACK ACHE

a)   Boil khal and then use it to massage the part applying a little force. Repeat for effective result.

b)   Rub original olive oil on the spot or back and drink 2 spoons of honey every morning

c)   Mix sandah oil, alum powder, lime juice. Apply on the part.

d)   A cuo of pounded carrot, a tin of sandah powder, a bottle of honey. 2spoons twice daily.

e)   Boil epo igi aganwo for 2day drink.

f)   Do hijamah.

BILHARZIASIS / SCHISTOSOMIASIS

A x parasite infection by a trematode worm acquired from infested water. It is a snail-borne water based parasitic infection caused katayama fever, blood-fluke. In Yoruba it is called **ATOSIAJA**

a)   Mix a cup of honey, 5 spoons lime juice. 2 spoons

b)   3 times daily

c)   Ewe epin, ewe osokotu, ewe asunwon. Squeeze all and later add lime juice.drink little by little.

BARRENESS

a)	Insert a small piece of thafar (hoof) bone into your vagina after your period.

b)	Recite all ayat ash–shifa in zaitun oil (1 bottle) and black seed oil (1bottle). A spoon morning, afternoon nyt. Fatia, Qursiyy, ikhlas and all other ayatush-shifa

c)	2l sidr leaves. Grind all & add plenty water. Recite ayate ruqyah in it. The woman will be drinking it very early in the morning & use it to bath in a clean place

d)	The person should be drinking shay-shayatlini, dunu-shayatlini. Rub her body with it.

e)	Ewe alipaida, ewe ailu, emo agbo, alligator pepper make all into powdery form. Use it to drink pap very early in the morning.

BODY PAIN

a)	Rub zaitun oil on the affected part of the body

b)	A spoon of saudah powder, a spoon of hulba, a spoon of garlic powder. Add to hot pap & take daily.

c)	Boil china gun powder tea in a cup of water. Filter, add to honey. Take it daily

d)	Ewe ipin, boil this leaves with pap water. Let it warm before drinking it. Morning afternoon nyt. You are to cook another at of leaves the second day.

e)	Boil pineapple leaves and drink.

BODY ODOUR

Use baking soda

BREAST (MORE FIRM, GROW BIG)

Crush bitter kola, aloe vera,olive oil, mixed with shea butter. Massage on your breast

BOBY AND FACE BEAUTY

a)	Mixed zaitun oil with lime juice. Apply on your body, leave for a while and wash it warm water.

b)	Mix carrot juice with coconut oil. Apply on your face and body. Wash after 30 mins

c)	Warm black seed oil for 3mins, allow to cool, add egg and a spoon of honey. Apply on your body & face.

d)   Mix all, olive oil, vinegar, sulphur, the fluid of ewe asunwon , fluid of ailu leaves. It cleanses and cure the following skin diseases; pimples, measles, pox, eczema.

TO BORN A BEAUTIFUL CHILD

During pregnancy, always drink luban zakar soaked in water and use luban incense burn on charcoal fire.

BAD VOICE (CRACK VOICE)

a)   Always lick honey.

BLOOD PROBLEMS /BLOOD DEFFICINECY:

a)   Always add zaitun oil to your food and rub on your body

b)   Always eat dates and honey

c)   Boil a mixture of tinni powder and nasit in water, drink it morning and evening

d)   Get juice of pumpkin leaves (UGU) mix with aloe vera juice. Add honey or milk. Twice daily.

e)   Eat bitter leaves raw.

f)   Squeeze cassava leaves and add honey.

g)   Squeeze poroporo baba, add powdered milk.

BLOOD LOST IN A CUT

a)   Wash the cut and apply olive oil. Bandage it and add olive oil.

BLOOD CANCER

a)   A tin of garlic powder, zaitan al, a bottle of honey. A spoon after your meals. Take carrot juice mix with honey

b)   Mix camel milk with camel urine a spoon each.

OBSOLETE BLOOD

Juice of bitter leaves, aloe vera juice pound carrot take 2 spoons, twice in a day

BREAST CANCER

a)   Mix 5 cups of aloe vera juice, a cup of honey 3 spoons, 3 times daily

b)   Pound aloe vera juice and rub on your breast wash it off the next day

c)   2 tins of saudah powder, half litre of saudah oil, a tin of rashad powder, 2 litres of honey with the wax, a tin of garlic powder, a tin of ginger powder, poundn pineapple head and mix a cup of it, take it regularly

d)   Change your eating habit, and include fruit and water

e)   Fast in fruit and water for a week

f)   Drink zamzam water

g)   Add black seed oil with grape, drink regularly

h)   Eat ruman fruit with seeds, add 3 ruman oil with 1 spoon of honey

i)   Celery (2 litres) + ½ litres of honey + 1 litres of apple vinegar 10ml daily

j)   Start drinking olive oil

k)   Do hijamah (cuppings) for the person once weak

l)   1 aloe vera, 3 fresh ginger, 1 pineapple, 1 soursop fruit pound and mix all together, regular intake.

m)   Camel milk with camel urine. A spoon each

BREAST PROBLEM
LACK OR SHORTAGE OF BREAST MILK:

a)   Breast feeding mother should be washing her breast with khal water

b)   Boil yahnsun with saujdah seeds 5 spoons morning

c)   If milk does not come out at all. The mother should squeeze Sodom leaves (Bombom). Use it to wash her breast

d)   Do you know male pawpaw leaves? Squeeze the leaves and wash the mother breast with it

BEING AGGRESSIVE

 Drink zamzam always with intentions

BLACK TONGUE

a)   Wash your tongue with apple cider vinegar and take this:

b)   Epo- ora, lime orange, few tomtom soak for 12 hours take once in a day

c)   Unshell a snail and after washing the snail swallow the snail and drink that snail water.

CATTARRH AND RUNNING NOSE

a)   Eat 3 olive seed and two spoons of honey

b)   Mix two spoons of ginger juice, 3 spoons of garlic, 2 spoons of lime juice, and 2 spoons of honey, mix in half cup of warm water then sip it.

c)   Swallows garlic after each meal.

d)   Eat garlic and ginger raw drink, 2 spoons of honey

CONJUCTIVITIS (APOLO)

a)   Mix small amount of aloe vera jelly in clean water. Drop two drops into your eyes 3 times daily

b)   Put honey in a clean water. Drop 2 drops into the eyes 3 times daily

CATARACTS

a)   Add zaitun with honey add just small at the tip of your eye

b)   Aloe vera jelly should be added on your eyes

c)   Apply olive oil mixed with antimony morning and night

d)   Eat Iru (Locust beans) very well

e)   Add 5 piecces of bitter kola into water (Orogbo) use as eye drop

f)   Squeeze out tomatoes leaves. Use as eye drop

g)   Kole orogba's leaves, squeeze and put as eye drop

h)   Squeeze ododo ewe iyeye with lime juice. Use as eye drop twice daily

CONSTIPATION

a)   Take sanamakim into hot water and drink on an empty stomache

b)   Eat zaitun fruit

c)   2 spoons of rashad powder, half cup of onion juice, 2 spoons, four times daily

d)   Drink a spoon of khaltufa mixed in half cup of cold water

e)   A spoon of aloe vera juice, a spoon of honey half cup of water take

f)   Drink 2 spoons of lime juice mixed in half cup of warm water

g)   Mix orange juice with honey, with little water drink always

CHOLERA

a)   A spoon of garlic powder, a spoon of saudah powder a cup of tomato juice, add little salt take it all and to be repeated 2 times for 3 days

b)   Add lime juice in a cup of hot water, drink in the morning for 1 weeks

c)   3 spoons of salt and 1 spoon of sugar add a spoon of vinegar (Khal), drink as simple close

d)   Chop 3 wonderful kola, with holy basil leaves soak lime juice for 3 days, 2 spoons daily for children 1 spoon to be taken at 4 hours

COLD & SHIVERING

a)   Boil ewe laali, 2 lemon orange juice, garlic, ewe tea, ginger, cloves drink regularly

b)   Mix a spoon of khall in half cup of water drink 2 times daily

c)   Mix garlic powder, ginger powder, saudah powder, in hot drink

COARSE AND DRY SKIN

a)   Mix honey with egg, rub the part with it

b)   Pound aloe vera, rub the body with it and wash

c)   Always rub your body with a mixture of olive oil and honey

CANCER

Regular intake of garlic reduce all stages of cancer

a)   Eat a spoon of garlic, 2 spoons of honey, a spoon of saudah powder and 2 spoons okf sebib

b)   Pound a tube of onion, 5 succullent piece of turmeric, a bottle of honey, cup of carrot juice. A spoon 4 times daily

c)   Eat five pieces of garlic fruit, 2 medium carrots 3 times daily for 1 month

d)   1 aloe vera, 3 ginger, 1 pineapple, 1 *swosop* fruit peel and pound all mix together

e)   Squeez out elegede and drink, also for hiv positive

f)   Drink ewedu

CHEST PAIN

a)   A spoonful of khal water in warm water. Half a spoon for children

b)   Eat garlic, ginger and honey together

c)   Eat garlic with ginger

d)   Boil 4 onions, place them on your chest one after the other for some minute for it to cool repeat for 4 days

COUGH

The dest and back should be rubbed with black seed oil take 3 spoons of oil per day

a)   Drink original honey

b)   Grind bitter kola ,mix with cup of honey take it constantly

c)   A cup of khal, 2 spoons of lime juice, 3 spoons of ginger powder, 5 spoons of rumman powder, a tin of habbatu saudah powder, 1 litre of honey, a tin of garlic powder, 3 spoons, 3 times daily

d)   Eat bitter kola with tomtom

e)   A tin of garlic powder, a bottle of honey, a bottle of olive oil, 2 spoons four times daily

CONSTANT FEVER

a)   3 spoons of khal, 2 spoons of honey in a cup of cold water. Mix and take it 2 times daily

b)   Mix a cup of khal, 8 spoons of lime juice, a bottle if saudah oil, 1 bottle of garlic oil, a tin of hulba powder, 1 bottle of honey. 3 spoons, 3 times daily

c)   Boil laali (Henna) leaves with N20 sugar, drink constantly

d)   Soak kigellia (Pandoro tutu) in a pap water with N30 sugar, drink constantly, soak for 15 hours.

CHILDERN TEETH PROBLEM

a)   From birth give your child zamzam water. It eases teething problem in a child.

b)   Mix a cup of honey, 3 spoons of lime juice, 1 spoon, 2 times daily

c)   Mix a cup of garlic water, a spoon of lime juice, half cup of honey, a spoon, 3 times daily

CONVULSION

a)   Pound two onions (White), five cloves of garlic, 2 ginger, a cup of honey, pound all together, mix all and take 2 spoons two times daily

b)   Kafura pelebe, kanfo rogodo, red oil, shea butter, palm kernel oil, mix all use to rub his/her body

c)   Give the child camel urine or black seed oil

CHICKEN POX & SMALL POX (MEASLES)

a)　　　Mix palm oil or palm kernel oil with honey, rub the body with it

b)　　　Mix aloe vera with honey, rub the body with it

c)　　　1 orange, 1 lime mix the juice with a spoon of garlic powder, take before breakfast.

d)　　　Mix rashad powder, a cup of khal, a cup of carrot juice, saudah powder (a tin), 3 spoons hulba powder,1 spoon of sitir leaves, 3 spoons of lime juice, 6 cup of honey.2 spoons, 4 times daily.

e)　　　Mix all zaitun oil, sulphur, fluid from asunwon leaves, fluid from ailu leaves, khal water. Use it to rub the body

f)　　　Grind bombom leaves + black soap. Use to bath

CHILDREN DIARRHEA

Pound carrots, add 1 litre of water. Heat it will light fire, sieve it and add little salt. Give it to child frequently

CHILDERN EXCESSIVE CRYING

Give him or her zamzam water to drink

CASTING OUT DEMONS

a)　　　Mix Luban, Haltiti powder, Ruman, Kajiji, Kisdul hind. Use them as incense. Take a mixture of zaitun oil, khaltufa, garlic oil

b)　　　Mix a handful of saudar powder, 2 spoon of haltiti, 2 spoons of saudah oil, 2 spoons of zaitun oil recite **Qursiy, Ikhlas, Falaq, Nas, fatia, A'mana rasul**, the last 3 verse of **suratul mumin** give him or her to drink.

c)　　　3 spoons of khal tufa, with 2 spoons of saudah oil. Add to half cup of water. Take for 1 month

d)　　　Do ruqyah.

CHOPPING FOOT

a)　　　A leaf of aloe vera pound and rub the affected part with it

b)　　　Mix zairun oil with pomade, rub the part with it

c)　　　Mix grounded alum, khal to form paste. Wash the part and apply the paste while going to bed. When you wake wash it with khal only.

d)　　　Mix khal tufa with honey. Apply

CEASE MENSTRUATION (MENSTRUATION THAT STOP)

a)   Camel Urine, Khal tufa, oyin ogidi mix all. 4 spoons morning & night 10 days.

b)   If it is spiritual eat 7 sidr leaves 10 days

c)   Boil yansun well a cup twice

d)   Khal (50cl), small murot, omi osan (4), 2 spoon saudah oil. 5 spoons, 3 times, 3 days

e)   Igi ato.Get the bark of this tree, soak it with water and sugar for 3 days. 3 spoons before food in the morning

f)   Iye aluko, ikode aiyekoto, poroporo oka baba, iyo, osun buke, ewe owu, epo amuje,egbo oruwo, egbo laali blend and grind it all. 2 spoons with hot pap

CURE TO IRREGULAR MENSTRUATION

a)   Take 4 spoons of honey, 4 times daily

b)   Garlic, Ginger, Turmeric, Epa ikun, Alubosa, soak all with water and add vinegar. 2 spoons morning and night

DIABETES

Do you know? Water leaf juice prevent diabetes, hypertension

a)   Drink Guava leaf tea for 3 month

b)   Stop eating starchy foods. Mix a tin of rumman powder, 1 bottle of saudah oil, 17 spoons of lime, 1 bottle of honey, a cup khal, 3 spoons morning alone

c)   A cup of pounded cabbage leaf, guava leaf, tin of hulba, a tin of garlic powder, pound a bulb of onion juice store and take 2 spoons before breakfast

d)   A tin of saudah powder, a tin of rashad power, half tin rumman powder, 3 spoons of murrat powder, 2 spoons of the mixture in warm water.

e)   Plenty sayad powder. Add 1 spoon of the powder to a cup of hot water allow to cool &drink 2 times daily.

f)   Mix a spoon of aloe juice in half cup of water twice daily

g)   Grind (abeere) seeds, 30 pieces of the seeds will be grinded and 2 spoons of its powder to be put in the oat

h)   Mix 5 grounded bulb of onions, add to 1 bottle of honey. ! spoon 3 times daily

i)   Try to be eating smoked unripe plantain.

j)   Grind all abeere, ahun, seeds of water melon, a spoon of it in oat very early in the morning

k)   Root of plantain, pound it and add it to water to honey.

DYSPEPSIA (INDIGESTION)

a)   Half tin of garlic powder, 1 bottle of honey, 1 bottle of olive oil, 3 spoons daily

b)   Always take honey and garlic

c)   Fenugreek seed (10pcs) grind, grounded ginger, Holy basil (Efinrin) 1 litre of water. Pound all, mix all and add little water and sieve. A small cup morning and evening. Be taking pawpaw and orange

DIARRHOEA

a)   Eat garlic morning and night

b)   Boil Al-babunaj and take its water

c)   A spoon of saudah powder, a cup of tomatoes juice, half cup of honey, a spoon of garlic, a little salt. Take all 2 times daily for a week

d)   Buy #10 ogi (raw pap that has been turned into watery one)Mix with little water and drink

e)   Take gaari without sugar, soak and drink without sugar

f)   Macerate, Basic leaf, bitter, lapalapa pupa, sieve and drink 1 stainless cup 2x daily

DANDRUFF & HEADLICE

a)   After shaving, apply khal. Repeat everyday

b)   Mix grounded garlic, khal, zaitun oil. Store for 3days. Start applying

c)   After shaving, cut Sodom leaves (bombom) and apply the milk-like water on the head

d)   After shave, mix olive oil, vinegar, fluid from ewe asunwon, fluid from ailu, Sulphur .apply on the spot

DIZZINESS (OYI OJU)

Ota inu iroko, iyere. Grind and mix all, use to drink hot pap

DEFFICIENCY OF BLOOD

a)   Boil a mixture of tini powder, nasit in water. Drink morning and evening

b)   Add zaitun oil to your food and rub on your body

c)   Get the juice of bitter leaves, mix with aloe vera juice. Twice daily, you may add milk or honey

d)   Eat the leaves of bitter leaves with holy basil very early in the morning for a week

DEWORMING

a)   Some back of neem tree (Dongoyaro) 6 lime oranges, cook for 10 minutes, until water changes colour. Allow to cool before drinking. A cup morning and night. 3 days for all ages

b)   Mix grounded corriandar seeds with khal

c)   Take sanamakin

d)   Lime juice + garlic paste a spoon daily not for below two years

DETOXIFICATION

Always eat food and drink water very early in the morning before eating anything in the morning and that is water therapy. Medically, it is unanimously agreed that WATER THERAPY alone when properly used could cure the following deadly diseases: Hypertension, stroke and a host of others.

DIFFICULTY IN SNEEZING

a)   Rub sanna on your nostril

b)   Rub rose on your nostril

c)   Chew ginger very early in the morning

d)   Eat saudah seeds everyday

e)   Crush black seed into powder, rap in cloth and bring to the nose for breathing.

DRY SKIN, FACE (COARSE SKIN)

a)   Mix honey with your cream

b)   Mix honey with egg, rub the coarse part with it

c)   Rub with zaitun mixed with lime

d)   Rub your body with aloe juice.

EPILEPSY

a) Do hijimah for the person

b) Take a cup of honey every morning for 1 week

c) Mix 5 spoons of harmol, 5 spoons of garlic powder, 5 spoons of saudah powder, half cup of khal tufa, a bottle of honey. Take 2 spoon of garlic oil before breakfast, then take 3 spoons of mixture after breakfast

d) Always drink zam zam with intentions

e) Mix a cup of aloe vera, a cup khal tufa, 2 cups of honey,2 spoons of luban zakar, 2 spoons of zukar nabat, 3 spoons , 3 spoons 3 times daily.

f) Always eat garlic with sebib after each meal.

g) Do ruqyah

h) Ahun, botuye, akoto, ewe taba. Cook all with water half cup. Morning and night for 2 months

i) Lady mantle, mistle toe, garlic, umbrella plant, salt. pound all, add salt and infuse in boiled water, allow to cool sieve 1 cup 3 times daily.

j) Squeeze the root of plantain, 2 spoons daily twice.

ELEPHANTIASIS

a) Epo akanya, epo akanmu, cook with water and drink, also use to bath.

b) Egbo ifon, ahun, eru Alamo grind all with black soup use to rub the leg

c) Abeere (to be taken in the morning), Ejinrin (to be taken at night). Grind wonderful kola very well, add aboniki rub, and rub the leg with it

d) Egbo ipetga, egbo igbesi, epo aganwo, egbo ifon eru alomo, alubosa elewe, olsan wewe, aidan, eru awonka, ,ewe odundun, ejinrin cook and drink very well'

e) Efo tete, koun bulala, obi infun boil and drink well. DO Hijamah on the head for the person for four weeks. That will be four time in a month, for second month, hijamah at the back for third month, hijamah on the leg.

EYE SCRATCHING OR BRINGING OUT PUS

a) Squeeze out water onions, add honey use as eye drop.

b) Mix rose water, zaitun, honey 50ml of the mixture. Put on your eye.

EYE PROBLEM

The prophet Muhammed (saw) said "The best of all eye medicines is antimony". It glorifies the sight and makes the eye lashes grow. It strengthens the optical nerves and preserves the health of the eye. For eye problems, use ANTIMONY.

a)   For red eye, put honey in a clean water. Use as eye drop

b)   Eye ache and leucoma, apply olive oil mix with antimony, both in morning and night. Always rub black seed oil on the sides of the eye, take a spoon of the oil daily, and always apply eye led (khal-l-haromain).

c)   Mix antimony with honey and put two drop in each eye.

d)   Always take zaitun oil mix in water, and rub the side of the eyes with the oil

e)   Half cup of carrot juice, half cup of honey, half cup of garlic water. 2 spoons 3 times

f)   Eat locust beans very well for cataract.

g)   Mix aloevera jelly in clean water. Two drops in eye.

h)   Squeeze tomato leaves, use as eye drop

i)   Always use Qurfat and antimony for any eye problem.

EYES FAINT

Mix three spoons of honey, 1 spoons of saudah oil, and 1 egg fry with zaitun oil (Olive oil). Eat every evening. Always apply eye led mixed with zaitun oil on your eyes before evening.

EYE BLURRNESS

Put rose water in your eye. Always eat saudah seed. It will go

EAR PROBLEM

a)   Soak a cotton wool in a khal water, put the wool into the ear

b)   Put two drops of garlic oil into the ear morning and night. use cotton wool to block it, repeat a day interval

c)   Onion juice, garlic water, olive oil. Mix all, put 2 drops in each ear for 3 days

d)   Drop some lime juice into the ear two times daily

e)   2 drops of honey into the ear, cover with cotton wool

f)   Put 2 leaves of ABAMODA in hot water, remove the leaves & squeeze out the water. Put into the ear very effective. Use cotton wool with it.

ECZEMA (Rashes, ring worm, chicken pox, small pox, skin problems)
a)   Rub olive oil on the affected part
b)   Mix zaitun oil with khal. Apply after bath daily
c)   Burn garlic into ashes, mixed with honey, zaitun rub on the affected part
d)   Pound one onion, mix with honey, sulphur, salt. Rub on the spots
e)   Pound aloe vers, rub your body with it. Wash it of after 15 minutes
f)   Mix saudah oil, garlic oil, honey, zaitun oil. Apply on the body
g)   Mix rashad powder, garlic powder, saudah powder. Mix with hot pap and drink
h)   Put little khal in your bathing water and bath the spot with khal very well and rub saudah oil.
i)   Get ewe asunwan egba. Rub the leaves on the eczema. For a week. That is all.
j)   Mix all: Vinegar, Olive oil, Sulphur, get the fluid from asunwan, get the fluid from ailu leaves. Apply on the spot.
k)   Sulphur, broken bottles, gun powder, grind all and add palm kernel oil, apply often.

ENERGY (To regain energy).
a)   A spoon of garlic powder into a cup of milk, morning and evening. Use honey if there is no milk
b)   Mix 5 spoons of garlic powder, 1 spoon of saudah powder, 3 eggs, little salt, fry with zaitun oil. Eat with bread, daily for a week.

FALLOPIAN TUBE BLOCKAGE

Get plenty asunwon leaves, koun bulala, aidan onigun merin (Tetrapleura tetraptera), small khal water. Cut that aidan and soak all in 5 litres of water and add small khal for 3 days. 2 spoons morning and night.

FIBROID

(Surgical removal of fibroid, laparoscopic, myomectomy)For ovarian cyst, before you go for laparoscopic myomectomy, try these:
a)   White onions, garlic cut all into eva bottle and soak for 3 day.Drink half glass in the morning on an empty stomach and last thing at night.
b)   Blend onions, garlic, honey, lemon, a short 3 weeks morning and night
c)   Boil aidan for 30 minutes one cup morning and night
d)   Olive oil + lemon juice empty stomach in the morning
Mix all, 7 spoons of saudah powder, 5 spoons of haltiti powder, 7 spoons of

hulba powder, half cup of khal tufa, 1 litre mof honey. 3 spoons morning and evening. Drink khal (white) on it or hot water after taking it

e)   Grind wonderful kola, add lime juice for 3 days a spoon 2 times

f)   Fofo olokun (White inside), eru Alamo, epo cashew, soak for 3 days, a spoon morning, afternoon and night

g)   Sundry pandoro gbigbe (kigelia). Grind, blend into powdery form add kaun bulala of one third of pandoro powder. Use with lime orange or khal water and later drink warm water on it. Six months. It will shrink..

h)   Pandoro, Bara, ewe akoko, ewe iyeye soak with pap water for three days. A cup 3 times daily.

FACE AND SKIN PIMPLES

a)   Apply khal water (white or red), allow to dry, then apply habbatu saudah oil twice daily for 2 weeks

b)   Wash your face with black seed soap, dry it then apply black seed oil on the spot

c)   Burn garlic into ashes, mix with honey. Apply on the spot

d)   Mix grounded garlic with olive oil. Apply on the spot

e)   Pound aloe vera, rub your body with it wash after 15minutes

f)   Add vinegar with honey drink and apply on the spot

g)   Sulphur, broken bottle, gun powder grind all and add to p.k.o (palm kernel oil). Apply often

h)   Mix all, sulphur, olive oil, khal, fluid from ewe asunwan, fluid from ailu. Apply often.

FAT REDUCTION

a)   Grind efinrin (basil leaves), cucumber, ginger, 1 lemon orange, tea spoon of aloe vera juice, half glass cup of water. Grind and mix all together. Take before bed until you see the result.

b)   Boil guava leaves and drink for 3 month.

c)   A cup of warm, 1 lime, 2 spoons of honey, 2 spoons of grinded ginger, in the morning empty stomach

FIRE BURN

a)   Rub aloe vera jelly on the part 3 times daily

b)   Mix sandah oil, zaitun oil (olive oli); egg yolk, Apply the mixture on the spot.

c)   Wash the spot with khal & apply honey

FRACTURE

Get camel or cow marrow, cook it with onions to become stew sip. Always eat onions, garlic and aloe juice. The wound will quickly.

FORGET FULNESS

a)   Soak luban in water. Drink on empty stomach

b)   Mix luban zakar with zukar nabat. 3 spoons first thing in the morning with honey

c)   Boil na'na leaves with saudah powder, garlic powder. Drink the mixture with honey

d)   A tin of garlic powder, bottle of honey, bottle of zaitun oil. 3 spoons, 3times daily.

FINGER NAIL PAIN

Put the affected part into a lime to make a ring morning and evening.

FEARFULNESS

a)   Rub al- misk on your chest

b)   1 bottle of honey, 1 bottle of olive oil, half tin ruman powder. 2 spoons every morning. Always rub olive oil on your chest and body.

c)   Drink zamzam water with intention.

FORGET FULNESS (ITS PROTECTION)

Avoid the following:

a)   Eating too much food

b)   Eating food nibbled at by a mouse

c)   Exess griref

d)   Reading epitaphs

e)   Gazing at stagnant urine

FOR WAKING UP EARLY

Drink tea containing garlic always

FOOT POSION

Before applying the mixture, wash with vinegar mix all: gun powder, garlic, ashes, black pepper, and Black substance from battery. Mix all and apply on spot. DON'T DRINK PLEASE

GUM DISEASE

a) Add 4 spoons of khal in a cup of warm water. Add little salt. Rinse your mouth with it always

b) Add olive oil to warm water, rinse your mouth with it

c) Rub your gum with garlic

GONORRHOEA

a) A bottle of saudah oil, a tin of rashad powder, 1 cup of water. Boil for some minutes. 3 spoons four times daily

b) A cup of khal, a tin of garlic powder, 3 spoons of hulba, a cup of honey. Boil for some minutes. 2 spoons

c) Massage the lower part of your abdomen with hot water mixed with

d) Mix onions juice with honey and little lime juice 2 times daily

e) Mix camphor with honey. Lick with little finger.

f) Steam bitter melon with heat in a pot for some minute. Squeeze out the juice, add little alum with raw egg. Drink repeat twice in a week

g) Soak bitter melon in water for three days with vinegar (khal water). Drink it little.

GENITAL HERPES

a) Iyalode funfun leaves, grind and mix with local soap use to wash the part

b) Grind these three leaves, mix with local soap, use to bath: iyalode funfun, ailu, asunwan egba

c) Mix vinegar, olive oil, squeeze ailu leaves, squeeze asunwan egba leaves, squeeze abamoda leaves add honey, aloevera juice. Mix all and rub the part with it.

HORMONAL IMBALANCE

Boil guava leaves + ginger. Drink very well a cup twice daily.

HAEMORRHOID (CHRONIC PILE JEDI, IDI TOYO)

a)   2 bitter cola, 2 red onions, 3 liters of water. Grind the cola and cut the onion, add 3 liters of water , boil and consume lukewarm, 3 times daily

b)   6 cloves of garlic, mango leaves, mango bark, 4 litres of water, boil all for 30 minutes and drink 3 times daily for 3 weeks

c)   After visiting toilet, mix 3 cloves of grounded gabrlic with palm oil and rub your anus with it

d)   Use omi iru (locust beans water). Boil omi iru and seat on it

HAIR LOSS

Cut two aloevera into cubes, extract two onion juice, 1 cup of coconut oil, if you can see chebe powder. Add it, rub your head with it.

BROKEN HAIR

a)   Add chebe powder to your cream

b)   Olive oil, honey, same quantity, warm it and apply it apply on hair, after 15 minute wash with warm water

HEPATITIS B

a)   Sundry eyin olobe (stone breaker) and make into powder use it to drink lipton tea without sugar

b)   Moringa leaves, garlic, ginger, turmeric, iyere (Black pepper) onions, habatu saudah powder, 1 lemon (cut into it), leaves of lemon grass, phyllantus amarus (eyin olebe) onion, cook all. 2 shots of cups morning and night.

c)   Do hijamah under your right breast. That is where your liver is. Hijamah must be twice in two month

d)   Cook enyin olobe and the person should be drinking it for 1 month in an empty stomach

e)   Epa ikun, Bara, Aloe vera, isu baka, 2 onion unripe pineapple, wonderful kola , turmeric, bitter kola. Blend all with squeezed bitter leaves water. Morning and night

f)   Pound 3 onions, add two litres of water and boil a cup daily for 3 weeks

g)   Drink 2 spoons of camel urine every morning

h)   Pound a cup of carrot,. Add water to it leave for 3 days, filter iot and add 3 spoons of lime rub the affected part with it

i)   Slice two onions, a spoon of saudah powder, fry with olive oil. Eat with camel milk powder

j)   Eat avocado

HYPERTENSION

 a)   Pound plenty garlic, olive oil (1 bottle) a tin of rashed powder, half tin of saudah powder, a spoon of sidr leaves powder, half tin of ginger powder, a cup of khal, 1 litres of honey. 3 spoons, 3 times daily.

 b)   Boil Nana leaves with water very well, add two spoons of khal, 3 spoons of honey, mix and drink, drink till condition improve

 c)   7 spoons of ruman powder, 1 bottle of garlic oil, 11 spoons of lime juice, 1 bottle of honey, half bottle of zaitun oil (olive oil), 1 bottle of saudah oil, 3 spoons of ginger powder, a cup of khal, boil Na'na leaves and add half cup. Mix all, 3 spoons, 3 times daily

 d)   Snail fluid, grounded garlic, garlic oil drink 2 spoons morning, afternoon and night

 e)   Epo igi ahun (astonnel bonnie), ata bawa (shombo) (cayenne pepper). Drink with water and add khal water (vinegar) for preservation for 3 days drink very well

 f)   egbo asofeyeye, raw garlic, small khal tufa soak for 3 days, small cups

 g)   Abamoda leaves (resurrection plant). Put 3 of these leaves in hot water for some seconds, remove and squeeze out its water, drink, 2 spoons morning and night

 h)   Cook abeere,alubosa elewe leaves and drink very well

 i)   Alubosa elewe, garlic, orogbo tutu (bitter kola) grind all and put into honey 3 spoons 3 x daily

 j)   Pandoro (kigellia), garlic, kafura pelebe cut and soak pandoro in water with the garlic for 3 days, drink very well

HIGH BODY TEMPERATURE

a)   Shower with cold water, take a spoon of saundah oil and rub body with it

b)   Squeeze bitter leaves with salt without water add original honey. 3 spoons, 3 times daily

HEART PALPITATION
Boil red jetropha leaves (lara pupa) with alum for 15 minute, later add honey and olive oil and drink

HEART DISEASES/ PROBLEM

a)   Mix one spoon of sitr powder, 1 cup of khal tufa, a bottle of zaitun oil, a cup of honey. 3 spoons 2 times daily.

b)   Seven spoons of zamzam and honey every morning. Say the intention of zamzam

c)   1 bottle of saundah oil, 1 bottle of honey, seven spoons of ruman powder, a cup of khal, 3 spoons in a day

d)   Eru ela, koun bulala, egbo sapo. Cook very well later put honey and cook.

SHARP PAINS IN THE THORAX

a)   Mix to spoons of honey with warm water drink before breakfast

b)   A tin of garlic powder, a bottle of honey, a bottle of olive oil, 3 spoons 2 times daily

RISING AND FALLING OF BLOOD PRESSURE
Drinking honey with garlic powder after dinner till you see changes

HEALTHY BREAST MILK

a)   Breast feeding mother should be drinking tea , hot pap

b)   Breast feeding mother should be wasting her breast with khal

c)   Breast feeding mother should rub her breasts with saudah oil and take its powder with hot pap

BREAST MILK THAT STOPPED

a)   Breast yansun with water and saudah seed, she is to eat saudah seeds and later drink the water with it

b)   Get bombom leaves (Sodom apple leaves), squeeze it

c)   Get male pawpaw leaves, squeeze the water rub your breast with it and drink little

d)   Wash your breast with khal, and wash her breast with saudah oil

HOUSE PROTRECTION

a)　　　　　Always play suratul Baqarah in your house

b)　　　　　Read suratul safat

c)　　　　　Put saudah powder in charcoal fire, the smoke will drive them away. God willing

d)　　　　　Read your adhkar morning and evening

HUNCH BACK

Rub zaitun oil and always take it

HICCUP

a)　　　　　A spoon of hulba, 4 spoons of khal, a cup of water and boil for 10 minutes, 3 spoons before bed

b)　　　　　Boil Na;na in water, mix a spoon of garlic powder with half cup of Na'na water rub our stomach with garlic oil mixed with zaitun oil

HEADACHE (MIGRAINE)

a)　　　　　Boil Na'na leaves with zamzam water, cool it and drink

b)　　　　　Put khal water in hot wter, drink and rub your head with it

c)　　　　　Warm habatu saudah oil, tie a little scarf on your head, put the oil on your head and drink a little

d)　　　　　Wash your head with zamazam water

e)　　　　　Bouil cloves (kanafuru) with yansun and drink

f)　　　　　Add khal water with zaitun, mix very well use to rub your head and drink

g)　　　　　Rub the part with garlic oil and always swallow garlic

h)　　　　　Mix half cup of zamzam, a spoon of sidir, eleven spoons of khal, pour into warm water, wash your head first and later wash other part of your body. Then apply saudah oil on your head

i)　　　　　Pluck ewe ariwo orun, squeeze the leaves and place on tour fore head

j)　　　　　Soak epo igi ahun, ata ijosi, soak for 3 days with water and vinegar. Drink for 7 days

k)　　　　　Put wonderful kola on your head

HIV&AIDS

a)   Form the habit of taking a spoon of black seed oil into hot water very early in the morning before food

b)   Oregano oil, Black seed oil , turmeric oil. Get all in same quantity. A spoon morning and night

c)   Pineapple, ewe agatu, eww asunwon, eru Alamo, aidan,, ewe igbo, boil all together, small cup. 3x daily

d)   Egbo awogba arun mejeji, egbo ifon, egbo eruju, eso asunwon, dry and pound all in powdery form, use 3 spoons 2x daily

e)   Do hijamah

INTERNAL HEAT

a) Soak a tin of rashad a powder, in a cup of water for 2 hrs. add a spoon of lime, 2 spoons of saudah oil, 2 spoons of olive oil, 2 spoons of lump sugar (zukar nabat) Drink all repeat for 3 days

b) Grind garlic with honey, 4 spoons 3 times daily

c) Ewe rinrin, ewe ibepe boil with water and drink

INTERNAL PAIN

a) Mix a tim of garlic powder, a bottle of honey, a bottle of zaitun oil, boil for 10 minutes, 3 spoons daily

b) Boil onion, lime juice with water, add alittle salt and drink

INFECTION

a) Drink guava leaves tea, boil the leaves and drink

b) 1 spoon of khal tufa, 1 spoon of cinnamon, dilute with water, to be taking an empty stomach

c) Tumeric, garlic, ginger, wonderful kola, cloves soak in water for 3 days with vinegar (khal) a little cup morning and night

d) Ewe epin, ewe osekotu, ewe asunwon, squeeze all   and mix with lime to be taken before food. A spoon

e) Always soak clove in a water and use it to clean after urination

f) Get a big garlic. Tie a rope to it and insert it in your vagina overnight remove the next morning

g) Add cloves with salt. Put in a warm water and sit on it

FOR CHRONIC INFECTION

Bara (bitter melon), epa ikun, kaun bulala, garlic, ginger, turmeric, cloves. Soak all with water and vinegar (khal) for 3days. 3 spoons morning and night

INSOMNIA

a) Crush garlic, 1 glas of milk, boil for 1 minutes, cool, add 1 spoon of honey take 30 minutes before bed
b) Mix honey with milk drink before bed time, boil panseke leaves and add honey, drink 1 hour before food or 1 hour after food
c) Drink original honey very well (Ata shombo) cayenne with water for 3 days. A cup 3 times
d) Epo igi asofefe (make it into powder and the person will take a spoon with water before bed
e) Boil ewe panseke and drink its water.

I DON'T ENJOY SEX WITH MY HUSBAND

a) Eat water melon
b) 1 tin of luban zakar, half tin of ginger powder, 1 tin of zukar nabat, nunu yougort, mix all the powder, put a spoon of the mixture into a cup of nunu yougurt morning and night

INFERTILITY

a) Get asunwon leaves in a large quatity, sundry and make into powder + half tin of cloves in powder + ¼ tin of iyere (African black pepper) + 200g of alum blend all and put 2 spoons in warm water before meal. Also for male , after the third day, make it every 2 days
b) Get 2 bara (bitter kola). Remove the hard back and soak with #200 pepsi drink for 3 days
c) Egbo sapere, aidan onigun merin, baka, alligator pepper, koun bulala, epa ikun, fufo olokun, iyere. Blend all together. A spoon in a day for 8 days before her menstruation. Boil akoko leaves and allow to cool for 12ours. Mix honey same quantity, a cup 2 times daily

JOINT PROBLEM

a) Mix lime juice, alum powder, saudah oil apply on the spot
b) Mix bottle of zaitun oil, a bottle of honey, 9 spoons of khal tufa. 3 spoons morning and evening
c) Apply zaitun oil mixed saudah oil. Massage well on the spot

d)   Boil khal (vinegar), massage on the spot with force regularly
e)   Taike 3 spoons of honey, morning and evening
f)   Do hijamah

JUNDICE (IBA PONJU)

a)   Take tulus water, 3 spoons, and every 3 hours for 24 hours. This is first step
b)   Haltiti powder, khal tufa, hulba powder, little sugar. Warm very well with water, let it cool, 3 spoons morning and evening
c)   Boil nasil like tea, put it down, add 7 spoons honey, khal tufa. 3 spoons 3 times daily
d)   Always add dawahul yaom to all your food
e)   To cure jaundice, unripe pawpaw, cut into smaller unit and boil with corn water (omidun) with little potash. Drink very well with eyin olobe (phyllantrus amarus)
f)   Boil buzuril fuJul and drink its water
g)   Cucumber (peel cucumber and boil the peeled ones and drink very well for 3 days.

KNEE PAIN

a)   Add 2 spoons of khal tufa (apple cider vinegar) in two cups of water sip throughout the day.
b)   Add 2 cups of khal tufa in hot water soak the knee in it.
c)   Boil grated ginger in a water for 10 minutes, sieve it and later add honey & lemon juice to it.
Drink 2-3 times a day.
d)   Freshly grated ginger and turmeric boil for 10mms & later add honey to it.
e)   Wrap few ice- cubes in a thin towel and place over the knee for 10-20mins repeat 3-4 times daily.

KELOID

Wash it with scent leaves (grounded) added with khal water. After washing, add this. Pound potash into powder, white from pawpaw tree, aloe juice. Add the mixture.

KIDNEY PROBLEM

a) You can prevent kidney problems. Take garden eggs leaves boil, cool and drink the water.

b) We have kidney beans. They look like kidney ad when cooked and eat also assist effective functioning of kidney.

c) 3 spoons of zaitum oil daily

d) 2 spoons of khal tufa in a cup hot water 3 times daily

e) Pound unripe date nut, a spoon of the powder, 2 spoons of onion juice, a cup of fresh cow milk 2 spoon, 2 times daily

KIDNEY STONE

a) A spoon of garlic powder, a spoon of zaitun oil, a spoon of lime juice, a cup of nunu milk, a spoon every morning before breakfast.

b) A bottle of honey, a bottle of zaitum oil, a tin of garlic powder. 3 spoons daily

LOOSING ONE'S VOICE

Mix two spoons of honey, and a cup of water, boil it, drink all four times daily.

LOW BLOOD PRESSURE

A level of garlic powder, a spoon of zaitun oil after each meal]

a) Boil pounded ginger in a cup of water. After cooling, add a spoon of onion juice, 2 spoon of honey. Drink before going to bed, repeat until condition improve

LIVER DISEASES

a) A spoons of sandah powder, a spoons of ruman powder, a cup of water. Boil and cool. Later add 2 spoons of khal. Take it 3 times for that day. Repeat it the following day

b) 3 spoons of khal, 3 spoons of honey in a cup of water. Take it two times daily.

c) Mix khal tufa, little zamzam water, pure honey. Mix and drink very well.

d) Do hijamah (cupping) under your right breast & back

e) Boil buzuril fujul & drink its water.

f) Boil nasit, drink its water morning & night

g) Pound a leaf of aloe vera, 3 spoons of honey. Mix in half cup of water. Take it daily

h) 3 spoons of honey, 3 times daily for a month

i) Slice three limes, put them in a cup of hot water. Allow it to pass the night and drink it first the following morning for a month.

j) Holy basil's fluid, bitter leaf fluid, osan ija gain, honey. Mix all & drink very well.

LOW SPERM COUNT AND WEAK CELL (no sex while using)

a) Cut carrots and add guava leaves boil well and drink, no sex please and take a week off & later repeat

b) 30 bitter kola, 6 tins of galrlic, 2liter of honey. Grind all into paste & add the honey. 3 spoons 3x daily

c) Harmolu powder (half tin), 1 tin of habatu rashed powder, 3 tins of zukar nabat, 1 bottle of rose water, wara malu half liter, 1 liter of honey. Mix all and use within 15days 2x daily

d) Get the following and cook all very well: asunwon leaves 1bitter melon, sagere roots, isu baka, onion leaves, garlic, kaun bulala, after boiling a, cup 3x daily

e) Starch, local eggs of equal quantity. Sun dry and later add lump sugar of equal quantity. 2 spoons to drink pap

LEPROSY

a) 2 spoons of habbatu sandah powder, two spoons of henna powder, 2 spoons of zaitun oil a spoon of khal tufa, 5 spoons of honey, a little salt. 2 spoons of mixture 3 times daily. Also rub on the affected part.

b) Mix apple cider vinegar with honey & rub it.

c) Acalypha wilkesiana (lara pupa). Grind these leaves and use it to cook cat fish and eat it.

d) Egbo awogba arun, oje oro agogo , etu bon mix with soap and use it to bath it.

LAZINESS & SLUGISHNESS

A spoon of black seed oil with orange juice for 11days in the morning. You will see the difference yourself.

LABOUR (FOR EASY DELIVERY OR WOMEN IN LABOUR ROOM)

a) Drink half cup of honey

b) Cultivate the habit of eating seven dates every morning before breakfast during pregnancy.

c) Get a cup of zamzam, recite intentions of zamzam and then drink it

d) Mix na'na leaves (mint leaves) with two spoons of rose water and half cup of honey sip it

e) Boil yansun as tea. Add 3 spoons of rose water with 1 cup of yansun tea. Drink it she will put to bed safely.

f) Boil sitr leaves and hulba seeds with 1 cup of water. During delivery, give her 1 cup.

LUNG DISEASES

Take 3 spoons of original olive oil 3 times daily.

MOUTH DISEASE

MOUTH ULCER use for mouth odour (for small kids and adult)

a) Rub your mouth with garlic oil or original olive oil. Allow for 30 minutes, after 30mins, wash off with boiled and cooled luban zakar water. After washing, mix garlic oil with luban zakar oil and rub your mouth with it and leave. Morning and night. It could be used for kids too. To get luban zakar oil, just buy olive oil and soak luban zakar in it for 2days. That is your oil

ALSO FOR KIDS

a) Soak cowries in lime water for 3 days, use to rub the kid's mouth
b) Use ewe ogbe ori akuko

MOUTH ODOUR

a) Mix cloves with honey, take a spoon morning and night
b) Mix powdered cinnamon with honey, a spoon morning and night
c) Brush your mouth with mixture of lime juice mix with honey in half cup of warm water three times daily Repeat for 3days
d) Use miswak to brush your teeth
e) After dinner, form the habit of eating cloves (kanafuru) with garlic and honey. A spoon of the mixture daily

PALATE AND TONGUE ACHE

Mix a spoon of honey with 3 spoons of lime juice, rinse your mouth with it 3 times daily

GUM DISEASE

a) Mix olive oil with warm water and rinse your mouth with it
b) Rub your gum with garlic oil after oil after a while, rinse your mouth with warm water that was used for boiling luban
c) Rinse your mouth with khal water, put 2 spoons of khal water in warm water

TOOTH CARE (TOOTH ACHE) AKOKORO

a) Rub garlic oil by the tooth side
b) Mix a spoon of cinnamon powder with 3 spoons of honey. Rub by the teeth side. Always gargle your mouth with khal water (white vinegar) before putting the honey and cinnamon
c) Boil olive fruits, boil it and inhale the steam of the water
d) Apply grounded garlic mixed with khal water on the paining spot
e) Rinse your mouth with khal water mixed with warm water, add a little lime juice
f) Uproot gbegi plants, add potash and cook. Add little to the spot

MUCUS

a) A spoon garlic powder, 3 spoons of honey to half cup of warm water. Drink the mixture every morning
b) Mix 3 spoons of honey in a bowl of hot water, cover your head with a towel and inhale the steam
c) Mix all 3 spoons of garlic, half bottle of honey, 5 spoons of olive oil. 2spoons, 3 times daily
d) A spoon of stiir, habatus saudah powder, half bottle of honey. 2 spoons, 3times daily

MUMPS & GOLTRE

a) Rub the spot with garlic oil
b) Mix a spoon of garlic powder with warm water and drink
c) Boil 3 spoons of khal water in a cup of water, Take everyday
d) Avoid anything cold, cold water, cold place
e) Pound garlic with your teeth and hold for 5mins before swallowing

MENTAL PROBLEM

a) Give him or her 3 spoons of honey, 4times daily
b) Allow bees to sting him or her two times daily

MISCARRIAGE

a) A spoon of honey, a spoon of habatus saudah powder, a cup of camel daily` Cook all lime oranges, garlic powder, habbatu saudah powder and Later add 2 spoons of honey morning and night

MALARIA & TYPHOID (TYPHISALMONEDA)

a) Mix 3 spoons of lemon juice, 3 spoons of honey in a cup of warm water. First before breakfast and lastly before bed

b) Rub your body with garlic oil

c) Always drink plenty water 30mins before food and water very well after your food

d) Unripe tomato (10), 7 carrots grind all add 7 bottles of water and 1 bottle of honey, small cup 3 times daily to give him strength.

e) 21 pieces of lime, scent leaves, cut the lime into two. Boil very well and drink half glass cup. Someone with ulcer must not take it.

f) Boil all, lemon grass, ewe oruwo, orange peel, pawpaw leaves, bitter leaves, scent leaves, a cup 3 times daily.

g) Boil henna leaves with #20 sugars. A cup 3 times daily

h) Soak kigelhia (pandoro tutu) with corn water and 2 spoonful sugars, a cup 3 times daily. Tested & Trusted.

MENSTRIAL PAINS

Buy 5 wonderful kola, soak with lime orange for 3 days. A spoon morning and night. Not for ulcer patient. Don't take it five days before your menstruation. Eat very well using it

MENSTRUATION COULD NOT STOP

a) Habatu saudah powder,1 bitter melon (bara). Boil the two together. Add honey to it. 3 spoons 2x daily

b) Grind some cloves, add with coconut oil and later add grounded charcoal to it. Half cup in a day

MUSCLE (WEAK MUSCLE) WEAK ORGAN CELL

Locate the veins to the affected part sting it three times, 3 times per week until there is improvement

MEN ABDOMINAL PROBLEM

a) Two spoons of honey, 3 times daily

b) Boil 3 onions and add a spoon of khal tufa, take all in a day. Repeat every day

NASAL

a) Crush black seed into powder, rap in a cloth and bring to tnhe nose for breathing. It can also cure any

b) Mix onion juice with khal. Soak into cotgton and put into your nostrils

c) Soak cotton wool into a lime juice, drop some of it into the nostrils

NIGHT MARES (BAD DREAM)

a) Get a spoon of black seed oil, 3 spoons of honey. Recite Qursiy and take before bed

b) Recite qursiy, iklas, falaq and nas and rub your body with it after blowing your palm

c) Pour little sidr water in your bathing water but never bath in the bathroom but a clean place

d) Burn them on charcoal black Ajiji, saudah powder. Haltiti powder. Always perform ablution before bed

NETTLE RASH

i. Egbo igi (grind) and add 1 bottle of lime juice. 1 spoon morning and night, after food, ulcer patient don't go near

ii. Grind 3 wonderful kola with 25cl of water drink 3 spoons, 2 times daily

OPEN SORES

Mix aloe vera juice with honey, use to form a paste on the sore.

POISON

a) Pound 6 bitter kola. Add 1 bottle of palm kern el oil, 5 spoons of honey, a cup of milk, mix and drink very well.

b) Chew aloe vera leafs constantly

c) Eat seven dates, and take 3 spoons of olive oil morning before breakfast

d) A spoon of olive oil constantly

e) A spoon of garlic powder, 3 spoons of habatu saundah powder, a spoon of ginger powder, a bottle of honey, 3 spoons of the mixture in half cup of warm water. Drink

f) Take sanamakin on an empty stomach, before breakfast, later eat 4 hours later.

PROSTRATE DISORDER

a) Eat soft leaves of guava and drinks it's tea

b) Ripe pineapple, Bara (bitter melon), koun bulala pound all and extract the water, later add malt khal or malt. A shot daily

c) Grind saw- palmetto 50g to 40ml of honey. Mix well 2 spoons, 2-3 times daily until condition improves. Always take fruit & vegetables

d) Grind plenty seed of date palm. Grind to powder. Mix with honey, take 2-3 spoons 3 times daily

e) Grind ewe taba & akogun root, soak in water in some time & sieve out the water. Later add ororo malu. 1 glass cup a day

f) Squeeze ewe pale without water & drink

g) Squeeze pygeum leaves

h) Cook ginger& drink

i) Root of water leaves. Cook and drink

ADVICE

a) Make sure you fast. It is called autophagy. Maybe on Mondays, Thursday. It boost ur body

b) Don't do hijamah for someone with diabetes

c) Take water very early in the morning before breakfast.it curses countless number of diseases: like hypertension, cancer

d) When honey is honey is mixed with any herbs, that drug must be used 1hour before food or 1hour after food

e) Take bee injection twice a year. It cures countless ailments and diseases. Your liver, kidney, heart will be ok and your immune system will be sound

f) Do hijamah don't do it on Wednesday

PREGNANCY POSITON (baby in wrong position in womb)

a) Habatu saudah powder, honey, Na'na oil. If you can't get na'na oil. If you can't get na;na oil, get the leaves, make it into powder mix well with others. 5 spoons 3 times daily. By God's grace the baby will change to normal position.

b) She will be drinking 2 spoons of zaitum oil very early before food till she birth.

c) Give her ewedu to drink for 1 week.

d) Read Q7a vs last verse, Q4b vs 35 into zaytum and rub her stomach with it

I WANT TO GET PREGNANT

2 tins of black seed powder, 2 tins of hulba powder, 2 tins of buzuril fijul powder, 2 liters of honey. Wara rakunmi (wara malu). Mix all the powders, put 3 spoons of the mixed powders in a cup of wara malu drink before breakfast for 40days.

PROSTRATE DISORDER

Pawpaw leaves, Maringa leaves, Grava leaves, garlic, sour sop leaves. Pound with mortar takes juice extract 3 times daily for 3-6 month. Also good for fibroids, cysts and cancer.

PILE

a) Rub zaitum oil by your anus always

b) Add 2 spoons of black seed oil, 3 spoons of lime juice to hot water. Let steam heat to your anus for 10mins. Always take a spoon of black seed oil mixed with the powder and rub your anus with the oil.

c) Get red jethropa leaves, mint leaves (na'na leaves). Boil the two and drink well

d) Chop 10 pieces of wonderful kola, kafura, soda water. Add the wonderful kola to 1 liter of soda water with 1kafura. Adults 2 spoons, children 1 spoon 3 times. Check for constipation and Diarrhea.

PREVENTION OF GREY HAIR

a) Apply zaitum oil on your head always

b) Never allow rose water on your head

PNEUMONIA

a) At night always put a spoon of khal tufa in hot water before bed.

b) Eat garlic, ginger and drink honey.

c) Always eat garlic

d) Boil 4 onions; place them on your chest one after the other for some minute for it to cool. Repeat for 4 days

e) Rub your chest and back with grounded garlic.

PROBLEM OF THE URINARY TRACK

a) Drink a cup of water containing a spoon of khal always.

b) A cup of pounded carrot juice. 1 spoonful four times daily.

c) A tin of hulba powder, a tin of black seed powder, four spoons of ginger powder, 3 spoons of sitir powder, 3 spoon of garlic powder, 1 cup of khal, 1 liter of honey, 3 spoons every morning.

d) A cup of honey, 2 spoons of black seed powder, a spoon three time daily.

e) Mix half cup of coconut water wit half cup of honey. Take it 3 times daily.

PENIS EFFECTIVENESS

a) Mix an egg, 2 spoons of honey, half tin of milk. Take it every morning.

b) 2 spoons of black seed oil, 2 spoons of honey to be taken very early in the morning before breakfast.

c) Half cup of carrot juice, a tin of black seed powder, 1 tin of rashad powder, 2 spoons of ginger powder, a cup of khal, 1 bottle of honey . Get 3 spoon of it to 50ml of zamzam. Morning and evening. You may substitute carrot for dates.

d) Half cup of carrot juice, a spoon of pounded bitter cola, a spoon of black seed oil, half cup of honey 2 spoon 2 times

e) Rub garlic oil around your penis after first round when you have cleaned yourself.

f) Drink garri 10mins before sex.

g) Eat garlic and ginger with honey 30mins before sex.

h) Soak egbo asofeyeje with water and little khal for 2 days. 3 spoons 2 times

i) Make pan Doro (kigellia), alligator pepper into powder. Take a spoon with khal water.

Cook all; pandoro, tutu, eru Alamo, eru awonka, alligator pepper. Half cup 3 times daily warm before drink squeeze ejinrin (bitter gourd), scent leaves with khal water. Drink well soak in 7up root of bitter leaf, aloe leaf root, root inabivi leaf, root of asofeyeye

POLIO

a) Mix zaitum oil, habbatu saudah powder; khal tufa, massage the affected part with it. The victim should avoid cold water.

b) Mix a tin of garlic powder, a bottle of honey, a bottle of zaitum oil. Take it every day

c) Always add a spoon of garlic powder in the child's milk if you want to prevent your child

PARALYSIS AND STROKE

Whenever stroke strikes, the first three minutes is very important and you must not play with it. Get that person seated gently without any harsh movement. Get a clean needle put it on fire to prevent any infections. Pinch the tip of the ten fingers of the person affected and press out blood. This alone will prevent the paralysis of the hand and leg. If it takes away the tongue also, squeeze the person's two ears very well and also pinch with that same and press out blood. Then get these:

a) A cup of khala tufa, 5 spoon of black seed oil, two spoons of luban zakar, 2 spoons of buzuril fujul, 2 spoons of grounded garlic, a cup of honey, 2spoon, 3 times daily.

b) Mix a bottle of honey, a tin of garlic powder. 2 spoon four times daily

c) Soak astoniel bonnei with cayenne pepper for 3 days with vinegar (5 spoons) in a 5 liters keg. A cup 3 times daily.

d) Get garlic oil, snail fluid, and grounded garlic. Mix all 2 spoons 3 times daily.

e) Mix all: grind abamoda leaves, ewe ato, garlic, snail fluid. Use it to rub the affected part

f) Get ewe ato, eru awonka, shea butter first, followed by eru awonka, ewe ato leaves, cook with water. 1 cup 3x daily

g) Ewe lefu losun, white snail, iyere grind the leaf with iyere cook with white snail and eat

h) Make into powdery form, kole arogba leaves, 1 alllegator pepper, take with , lime orange

i) Bone marrow, 3 cloves,egg, garlic oil, mix all 2 spoons 3 times

j) Worowo vegetables, squeeze and add honey same quantity. 3 spoons morning and night mix with black soap and use to bath 2x

PROBLEMS AT EARLY STAGE OF PREGNANCY

2 spoons of honey before bed and first thing in the morning. When it is serious take it three times

PROLONG ILLNES

a) Put cold press black seed oil in hot water to be taken very early before food

b) Khal tufa(2 spoons), shiffa (2 spoons) into half cup of hot water.allow to cool and use nit twice daily

c) Get plenty scent leaves, osan ijagayin, boil very well, a cup 3 times

QUICK EJACULATION

a) Soak all bara (Bitter melon). Epa ikun, Akokoun soak for 3 days, a spoomn 3 times

b) Aidan toro, garlic, epo aganwo soak all folr 3 days. Small shot 3 times daily

c) Garlic (5), bitter kola (5), ginger (1), blend all with 1 litres of water. Add honey 1 shot 3 times before food in the morning and night

d) Coconut, plenty tiger nuts, dates (dabinu), water, watermelon, get the extract from coconut melon and tiger nut, add it to squeeze and melted Daten and later add small honey, 3 spoons 3 times

e) Drink garri 10 minutes before sex. It works

f) Eat garlic and ginger 30 minutes before sex and after first round use garlic oil to rub under your pennis

RING WORM

i. Apply undiluted khal tufa to the area with a clean cotton ball several times daily

ii. Apply aloe vera, leaves overnight and wash next day

iii. Mix vinegar with salt. Apply.

RUNNING STOMACH

a) Get fresh pap, add small water mix and drink it raw

b) Rub olive oil around your stomach

c) Take a spoonful of garlic powder mix with honey after every 2hour.

RHEUMATISM/ARTHRITIS

a) Boil honey well and later add. Locust bean (iru) while on fire. Put it it down and to cool 3 spoons 3x.

b) Boiled black seed oil to be mixed with blended (cayenne pepper (bawa). 1 spoon, twice daily. Boil another black seed, use it to rub the body & the spot

c) Turmeric, moringa powder, black pepper (a spoon), ginger, garlic, black seed powder, cinnamon (a spoon), others will be a thin each. 3 spoons, 3x daily.

d) Mix four spoons of carrot juice, half cup of fresh cow milk two spoons of honey. Drink daily for 2months.

e) Mix Al-babunaj with olive oil, boil together and rub the spot while still warm

f) Mix garlic powder, honey, hulba powder. Rub on the spot twice daily

g) Mix zaitun oil with black seed oil. Rub on the spot and do hijamah.

STOMACH ULCER
a)   Boil turmeric and add milk
b)   Mix habatu rashed powder with dried banana skin powder. Eat with fresh banana
c)   Take pineapple juice with honey
d)   Take shea butter.
e)   Soak pounded aloe vera overnight. Take it the next day 2 times
f)   Eat zaitun fruit with 2 spoons of zaitun oil before breakfast and before bed
g)   Cut into piece and soak. 3 unripe plantain and 6 okra. Soak for 3 days. 5 spoons 3x
h)   Soak all pawpaw into a 5 litre water. A cup 3times daily
i)   Soak cayenne (bawa) pepper and drink
j)   Squeeze orugo leaves.very effective

STOMACH ACHES
a)   Drink a spoon of garlic powder mixed with half cup of milk.
b)   Take honey.
c)   Drink 3 spoons of olive oil in half cup of warm water. 3x
d)   Squeeze bitter leaves add honey to be taken before dinner.
e)   Lime juice in half cup of warm water. Drink it first thing in the morning for 3 days.
f)   Soak 3 spoons of rashad powder in a cup of water, then add 1spoon of lime juice. Drink well. Repeat it 3x daily
g)   Drink khal water so far your stomach ache is not ulcer.

SKIN PROTECTION
Always rub your body with zaitun oil mixed with black seed oil.

SKIN TAG

a)   Apply khal tufa (apple cider vinegar) for 1 month
b)   Apply castor oil mixed with baking soda for 1 month
c)   Apply pineapple juice and wash in the evening.

SICKLER
a)   Cress seeds powder, black seed powder, garlic powder, honey. Mix all a spoon 3x daily. Adult 2-2- 2, child 1-1-1
b)   Get juice of pumpkin leaves, /ugu/bitter leaves mix with aloe vera juice. Twice daily. Add milk or honey

c)   Mix 1 orange, 1 line, an egg yolk, 3 spoons of honey. Take daily
d)   Pound 1 tube of garlic, 1 kilo of carrots, a tin of sabib,1 bottle of honey. 3 spoons daily.
e)   Take a spoon of garlic with a spoon of zaitun oil. After each meal

SWOLLEN BODY

a)   A spoon of ginger powder, a cup of khal, a cup of honey. 2 spoons 3x daily.
b)   Rub honey on the swollen spot. And a spoon of honey before breakfast and before your dinner
c)   A cup of honey, 5 spoons of khal. 3 spoons of lime juice, little salt. Boil a bit & use it to rub the swollen place when cool.

SEXUAL IMPOTENCY

a)   A cup of cow fresh milk with a spoon of garlic powder. Repeat for 1 month
b)   Eat date with onions & drink honey always
c)   After meals, eat fresh honeybee wax
d)   Boil half cup of onion juice with half cup of honey. A spoon after each meal.

SPERM COMING OUT OF WOMEN AFTER SEX (EDA OBINRIN)

a)   1 Bara (bitter melon), abeere 3malts. (Rush abeere and remove the back of bitter melon. Cut the melon and soak well the malt together with grounded abeere. 2 shots morning & night. If it disturbs, reduce to 1 shot. Add powdered abeere to shea butter and use to rub your vagina.
b)   Isu ewura pupa, 1 plantain, starch. 2 small st lous.sun dry all and grind. 2 spoon into pap.
c)   Ikarahun igbin, 1 allegator pepper. Grind all and take 2 spoons into pap and drink.

SIEZED FEACES

a)   Eat vegetable and take oranges and lot of water

TUBERCULOSIS

a)   Grind alligator pepper, little salt, a bottle of honey. Mix all and take 3 spoons 3times daily.
b)   Grind dried pawpaw seed, add a bottle of honey, mix take 3 spoons, daily
c)   A cup of khal, 2 spoons of lime juice, 1 spoon of ginger powder, 5 spoons of ruman powder, 1 tin of habbatu sandah powder, 1 liter of honey. 3 spoons, 3x daily

THROAT PAIN

After 2 hours, mix a spoon of khal, 2 spoons of honey in half cup of warm water and sip it.

TESTICLES & SCROTUM PAIN

Pound onions, add 5 cups of water half cup of khal tufa. Leave for 3days. Take it for 10 days.

TO BORN A BEAUTIFUL CHILD

During pregnancy, always drink luban zakar soaked in water when your pregnancy is around 7months.

TO STOP BLOOD LOST IN A CUT

Wash the cut and apply zaitun oil

TOOTH ACHE

a) Same quantity oregano oil, clove oil, mint oil drip it directly on the affected part.
b) 3 spoons of honey, 1 spoon of cinnamon powder dip it on the tooth

UNCONSCIOUSNESS

a) Give camel urine
b) Give habatu saudah oil
c) Rub musk into the nostril of the person
d) Hit k1 with biro. K1 is an accunpuncture term which beneath your feet

TO FEEL YOUNGER (AN OLD PERSON)

A tin of garlic powder, a cup of cow milk boil for 5 minutes, add 5 spoons of grounded ginger, ten spoons of za'faran powder, 6 spoons of black seed powder, 6 spoons of habatu rashad, powder, 6 spoons of yansun powder, 1 liter of honey. Mix together & store. A spoon before bed daily

TO BE LIVELY & HAPPY

a) Take 3 spoons of olive oil
b) A spoon of black seed powder, 2 spoons of khal, 1 spoon of sidir leaves powder4, a cup of water and drink always.
c) Form the habit of reading and listening to Quran daily

TO REGAIN WEIGHT

Take two spoons of olive oil twice daily

TO REGAIN ENERGY

a)   Mix 6 spoons of garlic powder, 2 spoon of habatu saudah powder, 5 eggs, and little salt fry it with a cup of zaitun oil. Eat with bread. Repeat for a week.

b)   A spoon of garlic powder, into a cup of milk. Take morning & evening. Honey could be a substitute for milk.

VEIN AND JOINT PROBLEMS

a)   Mix garlic with zaitun oil. Rub on your body morning & evening

b)   Take 2 spoons of honey every morning & rub on the spot.

c)   Boil khal and apply with a little force on the part. Repeat

d)   Mix lime juice, alum powder, black seed oil. Apply on the spot.

e)   A bottle of zaitun oil, a bottle of honey, seven spoons of khal tufar 3 spoons morning & evening.

f)   Apply zaitun oil on the affected part. Massage well.

VOMITING

a)   2 spoons khal, 2 spoons of zaitun oil, 2 spoons of honey. Heat for 1 minute. Take all

b)   Add a spoon of khal to half cup of water. Take it 3 times daily.

c)   Add zaitun oil to water. Take it

WITHLOW

a)   Ewe rinrin, shea butter, white beans. Grind all and mix with shea butter. Use to bandage the spot.

b)   Mix khal water with lime juice, dip your hand into it and allow for 10mins

WART ON THE SKIN

a)   Mix lime skin with khal and leave for 7 days. Filter and rub on the spot

b)   Scape it with razor and apply lime juice mix with khal.

WOUND (UNHEALED WOUND)

a)   Mix khal tufa (apple cidar vinegar) with honey apply on the spot and bandage

b)   Mix black seed oil with honey. Apply on the spot

c)   Wash the spot with zamzam mixed with little salt apply a/b above

WHOOPING COUGH

a) Eat olive fruit regularly and take 2 spoon of zaitun oil 3 times daily

b) Pound 2 white onions, 1 bottle of saudah oil, a bottle of honey. 2 spoons 3 times daily for 3 month

c) 2 spoons of garlic powder, half cup of honey, a cup of milk. Drink daily.

WEAK LIBIDO (SEXUAL WEAKNESS)

3 gingers, 3 lemon, 1 onions. Remove the skin, put in a blender & extract the juice. Take a glass every morning on an empty stomach for 2 weeks

YELLOW FEVER

a) Pound 5 onions, boil with 3 cups of water. Take a cup in the morning & evening

b) A spoon of haltiti powder, 3 spoon of khal tufa, 3 spoons of hulba, a cup of water, little sugar. Boil them. Half cup morning & evening.

c) Mix a tin of garlic powder, a bottle of honey, a bottle of zaitun oil. 3 spoon daily.

d) Add 3 spoons of olive oil with 2 spoons lime juice. Take before bed. Ulcer patient must not take lime juice.

WATERY SPERM

a) Get sayad powder. Turmeric powder, mix together put 1 spoon into a cup of water. Allow to cool and drink. 2x daily

b) Habatu rashad powder, garlic, habatu saudah powder, tulus water, honey (1 litre). Powder mix all very well and store for 12 hours. 3 spoons 2x daily.

c) 7 spoons buzuril fujul, 1 litre of honey. Mix well and be taking it 3 spoons 2x daily for both husband & wife

Honey + garlic powder. Mix the two before brushing take 3 spoons. It is for woman alone.

30 NATURAL ADVICE

1) Stay away from cold water. It close four vein in the body and may lead to liver problem.
2) Don't take garlic with drugs
3) Ulcer patient must stay away from lime juice, khal water, (apple cidar vinegar)
4) Pregnant woman should not use any prophetic medicine except honey unless you are told to do so or your pregnancy is up to $7^{1/2}$ month
5) Always use herbs 1 hours before meal or 1 hour after meal any herb that has honey
6) Make sure you fast twice in a week, it boost immune system
7) Don't do hijammah (cupping) for someone with diabetes
8) Always observe water therapy, It cure countless number of diseases.
9) Take bee injection, it make your body chemistry sound
10) Don't do cupping on Wednesday.
11) Don't breath in your drinking water
12) Do not drink khal first thing in the morning
13) Someone suffering from ophtalmia should not eat date
14) Too many onions being eaten raw may cause headache, affect intellect and make a person forgetful
15) If habatu saudah is grounded up with vinegar, mad into paste, rubbed on the abdomen, they kill intestinal worms
16) Figs relieve a chronic cough. Eat it
17) Don't always talk in the toilet you are only inviting disease to yourself by doing so
18) Always sleep with your right side
19) The best of all eye medicine is ANTIMONY
20) Aloe wood is the best for brushing teeth
21) Lemon cures diarrhea and palpitations. it remove ink stains from clothes, and freckles from face
22) Sniffing onions after taking medicine prevent vomiting.
23) Dates increase sexual power when combined with palm kernels
24) If a person who is suffering from ophthalmia eats dates, he will have headache and other ill effect
25) Figs relieve a chronic cough, act as a dimetic and clear blockings
26) Garlic acts like antidote for bites and scorpion sting
27) Carrot arouse desire for sex and produce good supply of semen
28) Black seeds cures all diseases except death

29) Cress seeds are remedy for tenesmus and activate semen
30) Fenugreek strengthens the heart

NAMES OF HERBAL LEAVES IN DIFFERENT LANGUAGES

ARABIC	ENGLISH	YORUBA	HAUSA	IGBO
Habbatu saudah	Black seed			
Asal	Honey			
Zaitun	Olive oil			
Zanjabil	Ginger	Ata ile funfun		
Ruman	Pomegranates			
Khal	Vinegar white			
Khal tufa	Apple cidar			
Khardal	Mustard			
Hinna	Henna	Laali		

ARABIC	ENGLISH	YORUBA	HAUSA	IGBO
Hulba	Fenugreek			
Habbatu rashad	Cress seads			
Jazr	Carrot			
Thum	Garlic	Ayu		
Tin	Fig	Apoto		
Tamar	Dried dates			
Basal	Onions	Alubosa		
Arak	Aloe wood			
Athmad	Antimony			
Atraj	Lemon			
	Cassia senna	Asunwon		
	Cow milk	Wara		
	Tetrapluera	Aidan onigun	Dawo	Oshisho
	Guava	Gurofa		
	Shea butter	Ori		
	Pawpaw	Ibepe		Abika
	Black pepper	Iyere		
	Pine apple	Ope oyinbo		
	Avocado pear	Ube		Ube - bekee
	Bitter lemon	Bara		
	Neam	Dongoyaro		Aghigh akom
	Fig	Opoto		
	Cashew	Kaju		
	Aloe	Eti erin		

ARABIC	ENGLISH	YORUBA	HAUSA	IGBO
	Guinea corn	Poro poro baba		
	Camwood	Irosun		Abosi
	Lime	Osan wewe		Oromankirisi
	Garlic	Ayu		Asoisi
	Bitter cola	Orogbo		Akialu
	Ginger	Ata ile funfun		
	Tumeric	Ata ile pupa		
	Basil	Efinrin		Nchuanwu
	Astoniel Bonnei	Ahun		
	Alligator pepper	Ataare		Osooji
	Bitter leaf	Ewuro		
	Resurrection plant	Abamoda		unwas

A-Z of Over 200 Diseases and Their Cures